Inside the pages of this book you will find herbal and nutritional strategies for relieving the inflammatory pain of:

- Osteoarthritis
- Rheumatoid Arthritis
- Gout
- Ankylosing Spondylitis
- Carpal Tunnel Syndrome
- Bursitis
- Neuritis
- Sciatica
- Tendinitis
- Lupus
- Lyme Disease
- Fibromyalgia

. . . safely, effectively and without the adverse side effects of prescription or over-the-counter drugs.

About the Author

CJ Puotinen has studied with some of America's leading herbalists and is a member of the Herb Research Foundation, the American Herb Association and the Northeast Herbal Association. In addition to magazine and journal articles on health and medicinal herbs, she is the author of *Herbal Teas, Nature's Antiseptics: Tea Tree Oil and Grapefruit Seed Extract, Herbs to Help You Breathe Freely* and *Herbs to Improve Digestion,* all published by Keats Publishing, Inc.

A KEATS GOOD HERB GUIDE

MEDICINE
21
CENTURY

HERBS TO RELIEVE ARTHRITIS

CJ Puotinen

Keats Publishing, Inc.   New Canaan, Connecticut

Herbs to Relieve Arthritis is intended solely for informational and educational purposes, and not as medical advice. Please consult a medical or health professional if you have questions about your health.

HERBS TO RELIEVE ARTHRITIS

Library of Congress Cataloging-in-Publication Data

Puotinen, C.J.
    Herbs to relieve arthritis / by C.J. Puotinen.
        p.   cm.—
    Includes bibliographical references and index.
    ISBN 0-87983-743-8
    1. Arthritis—Alternative treatment. 2. Herbs—
        Therapeutic use.
  I Title
  RC933.P86 1996
  616.7'22081—dc20   96-27547
                                                       CIP

Printed in the United States of America

Published by Keats Publishing, Inc.
27 Pine Street (Box 876)
New Canaan, Connecticut 06840-0876

98 97 96   6 5 4 3 2 1

Contents

HERBS TO RELIEVE ARTHRITIS

Introduction

The illnesses associated with inflammation have differences and similarities. Sciatica is caused by the inflammation of a nerve, rheumatoid arthritis is an autoimmune disease, osteoarthritis is the degeneration of weight-bearing joints, gout is caused by the buildup of uric acid in the body, carpal tunnel syndrome results from a nerve's compression, fibromyalgia (also called fibrositis) and lupus are inflammations of connective tissue, neuritis is an inflammatory disease of peripheral nerves, Lyme disease is a bacterial infection spread by tick bites, bursitis involves small sacs of fibrous tissue filled with fluid and ankylosing spondylitis is a rheumatoid disease of the backbone that can fuse joints. Their definitions and diagnoses vary, but all of these illnesses produce the same debilitating pain that prevents people from moving freely and living full, active, happy lives. They share another characteristic, too. All can be treated with nutrition and herbs with results that approach or exceed those of orthodox medical treatment, without the adverse side effects of prescription drugs or surgery.

That statement may surprise patients whose doctors have told them that inflammatory illnesses cannot be cured, prevented, reversed or slowed. Most American physicians agree with Robert Phillips, Ph.D., a psychologist whose book, *Coping with Osteoarthritis,* warns, "Is there any particular diet that is most appropriate for osteoarthritis? The answer is a resounding no!"

For decades the Arthritis Foundation denied the link between diet and arthritis, censoring anyone who suggested otherwise. While it is now conducting dietary research, its position on special diets and other "unapproved" therapies is still negative. The Arthritis Foundation upholds a philosophy of medicine that has prevailed in the United States for most of the 20th century. Doctors know best, patients should be protected from unapproved therapies, the only treatments a patient can choose from are those that have been officially endorsed and patients should be discouraged or prevented from experimenting on their own.

But if orthodox therapies worked, would people of all socioeconomic and educational backgrounds invest a billion dollars every year in alternatives? Orthodox medicine's failure to cure chronic illnesses like arthritis results from its failure to address the cause of disease. Western medicine is called "allopathic" because it treats symptoms with therapies that oppose those symptoms. It uses prescription drugs and surgical hip replacements to suppress or alleviate pain and inflammation, not to cure or reverse or prevent the disease itself.

In the treatment of inflammatory illnesses, millions of people around the world have experimented with what American physicians consider unusual, unorthodox, untested, unproven and unapproved therapies. Many have obtained good to excellent results—in some well-documented cases, total cures.

Obviously, not every treatment works for everyone, and this book does not intend to diagnose or prescribe specific therapies. But each of the following approaches has helped heal inflammatory illnesses, and, in contrast to prescription drugs and surgery, they are inexpensive and free of adverse side effects. They range from simple changes in diet to specific herbs or nutritional supplements, and they include short-term techniques that alleviate pain as well as long-term therapies that address the cause. Most of the therapies described here apply to all inflammatory diseases.

NOTES ON STANDARD TREATMENTS

Almost everyone who sees an American doctor for help with arthritis, rheumatism and related diseases is told to take aspirin. Aspirin is an anti-inflammatory drug; it reduces swelling, relieves pain and often allows the patient a wider range of movement. Because small, infrequent doses of aspirin lose their effectiveness over time, arthritis patients must increase the dose and frequency, often taking two or more aspirins per hour for pain relief. The *Journal of the American Medical Association* has reported that even small doses of aspirin can cause high or irregular pulse rates, swelling from fluid retention and albumin in the urine. Other side effects include nervousness, confusion, internal bleeding and the destruction of vitamin C in the body. Overdoses are fatal. Aspirin does not prevent, cure, reverse or slow the progress of arthritis, rheumatism, gout, ankylosing spondylitis, bursitis, neuritis, neuralgia or any other inflammatory illnesses; all it does is suppress pain temporarily.

Aspirin is one of several drugs called nonsteroidal anti-inflammatory drugs, or NSAIDs. These include ibuprofen, indomethacin, naproxen, piroxicam, phenylbutazone, sulindac and tolmetin. Like aspirin, these NSAIDs relieve pain and stiffness in many patients but they do not heal inflammation. Their side effects are numerous and often debilitating. One study showed that NSAIDs kill 2,600 rheumatoid arthritis patients per year and require 20,000 to be hospitalized. The U.S. Food and Drug Administration (FDA) attributes 10,000 to 20,000 deaths and an estimated 200,000 to 300,000 cases of gastrointestinal bleeding to their use every year.

Cortisone drugs are also widely prescribed for inflammatory diseases because they bring almost miraculous improvement to painful joints. Once considered a medical miracle, drugs such as prednisone, hydrocortisone, dexamethasone and other corticosteroids offer short term relief but their side effects include peptic ulcers, heart disease, osteoporosis and spontaneous fractures, mental disturbances, high blood pressure, damage to the liver and kidneys, diabetes and blood disorders. Like aspirin, cortisone drugs do not prevent, cure, reverse or slow the progress of any illness, so symptoms are often worse when the drug is stopped than they were before treatment began.

Gold compounds have been used in the treatment of arthritis since World War I and in 1960 they were proven to control the symptoms of rheumatoid arthritis. Gold can be taken orally or injected. Like aspirin and cortisone, gold does not cure, reverse or prevent rheumatoid arthritis; it suppresses symptoms by inhibiting cellular activity that contributes to tissue damage and inflammation. Because gold has potentially damaging effects on the kidneys, lungs, liver, bone marrow and skin, it is usually prescribed when the patient no longer responds to other drugs. Patients' blood and urine are routinely tested for signs of liver, kidney and bone marrow damage. Common side effects include diarrhea (oral gold therapy), skin rashes, painful mouth sores and decreasing effectiveness of the therapy.

Disease-modifying antirheumatic drugs or DMARDs are powerful drugs believed to slow inflammatory disease. Gold treatments belong to this category, as do hydroxychloroquine, chloroquine and penicillamine. Because they are slow-acting and require months of use before patients improve and because they are highly toxic and have dangerous side effects, patients taking these drugs must be carefully monitored.

Another allopathic approach to rheumatoid arthritis is the use of immune-suppressing drugs. Rheumatoid arthritis is an immune system disorder, and by slowing cell division and slowing the entire immune system, doctors try to slow the disease. Azathioprine, chlorambucil, cyclophosphamide and methotrexate are immunosuppressant drugs used in this manner. Patients must be supervised closely because of their increased vulnerability to common infections.

Antibiotics, not usually associated with arthritis, are actually important in the treatment of at least two inflammatory illnesses. The bacteria responsible for chlamydia nonspecific urethritis were shown to cause a form of unexplained arthritis in young women when nearly half of the tested patients had chlamydia bacteria in their joints. Bacteria transmitted by infected ticks cause Lyme disease, which produces arthritis symptoms in its victims. Antibiotics remain the preferred treatment for bacterial infections, especially if they are diagnosed early.

Once Lyme arthritis develops, usually accompanied by nerve problems, the illness no longer responds to oral antibiotics. Intravenous antibiotic therapy is of questionable value in advanced Lyme disease, for while physicians often claim the illness has been cured after weeks of this expensive, painful, time-consuming therapy, their patients display many of the symptoms they exhibited before treatment and are further debilitated by the antibiotics' side effects.

Food and Arthritis

Of all the "natural" approaches to the treatment of arthritis and other inflammatory illnesses, the most widely used is diet. Though most American physicians still discount their patients' observations that certain foods seem to cause swelling and inflammation, American researchers have begun to confirm what is common medical knowledge in other countries, and their reports in medical journals document the links between diet and inflammatory illness.

Dava Sobel and Arthur C. Klein published an extensive report of arthritis-related research in their book *Arthritis: What Works*, citing studies in which physicians measured significant joint swelling (as much as two ring sizes in fingers), pain, loss of grip strength, reduced range of motion and other symptoms of inflammation within hours of the patient's consumption of key foods.

One connection between joint pain and diet is obvious: most arthritis patients are overweight. Excess weight puts increased stress on weight-bearing joints such as knees and ankles, making movement even more painful than it would be otherwise. It is difficult for anyone on America's high-fat, low-fiber, refined food diet to lose weight, even if he or she is physically active. Add the sedentary lifestyle that accompanies the pain of arthritis and it's almost impossible. But when someone with an inflammatory disease makes significant dietary changes, both excess weight and joint pain can disappear.

In his early 20th century studies of primitive cultures, dentist-anthropologist Weston Price found whole cultures that not only had no tooth decay, misshapen dental arches or crowded teeth, they had no heart disease, cancer, tuberculosis, arthritis, rheumatism, diabetes or other chronic ailments. Yet when these same natives adopted the white flour, white sugar, refined salt and oils of modern civilization, their health decayed along with their teeth.

The native people who remained free of arthritis and other inflammatory diseases ate whole, unrefined, unprocessed food, much of it raw, from a variety of sources. This is in keeping with what we know about the evolution of human digestion. Human beings are omnivores. Our bodies are designed to consume and digest just about everything: all kinds of seeds, nuts, fruits, vegetables, meat, fish, eggs, roots, tubers—anything and everything that's edible.

Most Americans, on the other hand, eat the same things every day. We may think we're eating a variety of foods but in most cases it's just different combinations of refined wheat, eggs, milk, potatoes and beef. Our meals are typically devoid of fruits and vegetables, low in enzymes, fiber and nutrients, high in fat, calories and toxins and as likely to generate modern illnesses as the white flour and white sugar that wrecked the teeth and health of Dr. Price's native tribes.

Nutritionists and researchers who specialize in diseases such as arthritis, rheumatism and other types of inflammation have found that a diet rich in variety and emphasizing fresh, whole, unprocessed ingredients, such as different types of vegetables, fruits, whole grains and cold-water fish, can be therapeutic.

According to Dr. Alfred Steinberg, an arthritis expert at the National Institutes of Health, fish oil not only is a proven anti-inflammatory agent, it acts directly on the immune system, suppressing 40 to 55 percent of the release of cytokines, which are compounds that damage joints. For decades, physicians scoffed at the alleged benefits of cod liver oil and other fish oils, which users described as "lubricating" arthritic joints. After medical journals reported multiple benefits from fish oils, marine supplements became widely prescribed, especially those rich in omega-3 fatty acids. Although marine oil supplements are still popular, possible nutritional imbalances from concentrated supplements have made whole fish a preferred source of omega-3 oils for many physicians.

Vegetarians have always claimed that meat consumption and arthritis go hand in hand. They're right. A 1987 Swedish experiment reported in the *Scandinavian Journal of Rheumatology* showed that a strict vegetarian diet improved the condition of more than half of the rheumatoid arthritis patients who followed it for four months. Twelve of the twenty patients aged 35 to 68 experienced less pain and better capacity when they excluded meat, fish, eggs, dairy products, strong spices, preservatives, alcohol, tea, coffee, refined sugar, corn flour and table salt.

In addition to animal fats, certain vegetable oils are suspect. Too much omega-6 type fatty acids can interfere with the body's assimilation of beneficial omega-3 oils; the most common offenders are corn, sesame, sunflower and safflower oils. Flaxseed oil contains over three times as much omega-3 as omega-6, giving it high marks, but most other vegetable oils contain little or no omega-3 and large quantities of omega-6. Even though their omega-6 percentages are high, canola oil, soy oil, walnut oil and extra virgin olive oil contain at least 1 part omega-3 for every 8 parts omega-6. In canola oil, the proportion is 1 in 2. Olive oil is considered a healthy choice because of its high percentage of monounsaturated fat. For those reasons, canola, soy, walnut and olive oils are recommended for cooking. Another supplement of interest to arthritics is evening primrose oil, which contains prostaglandin-interrupting gammalinolenic acid (GLA).

In *Food—Your Medical Miracle*, medical journalist Jean Carper described the experience of New Jersey physician Joel Fuhrman, M.D., in his treatment of a 62-year-old woman. The patient had severe rheumatoid arthritis and other medical problems and was taking nine prescription drugs. She had not been able to close her hand to make a fist for 10 years and had extensive pain in multiple joints.

Like most American physicians, Fuhrman knew it was "preposterous" to think that anything as simple as diet might help arthritis. Still, he was willing to experiment. The patient went on a medically supervised fast and her arthritis disappeared. Such dramatic improvements with fasting are so common that many researchers recommend short-term fasting for rapid pain relief and temporary remission of nearly all arthritic conditions.

After her supervised fast, Dr. Fuhrman's patient became a vegetarian. Fuhrman reported that five months later she was still on the vegetarian diet and free of symptoms.

The advantage of experimenting with one's diet is that it's easy and inexpensive. If going without certain foods will reduce inflammation and pain, the outcome is often apparent within days. Everyone's system—and illness—is different. The connections between diet and inflammatory illness are so well-established that anyone can explore them and expect at least partial relief.

Some people with arthritis are sensitive to members of the nightshade family, which includes tomatoes, potatoes, eggplant, peppers and tobacco. These plants contain solanine, a chemical that inhibits an enzyme which is active in muscle and joint movement. The nightshade elimination diet is controversial, but most arthritis researchers agree that at least some people—from one in three to one in ten—are affected by these plants.

Bell peppers and chili peppers, whether red, yellow, orange, white or dark purple, are all potential problems for the nightshade-sensitive and they can be found in paprika, some cough drops, barbecue sauces and even pain relief ointments. Potato starch, a thickening agent, can appear in unlikely places, such as yogurt and convenience foods. Many Middle Eastern foods make extensive use of nightshades, especially eggplant, and some spicy Indian dishes contain peppers and potatoes. If you suspect that nightshades cause your inflammation, read labels with care.

Among the nightshades, tobacco is a special problem and avoiding second hand smoke can be a challenge even if you don't indulge yourself. If you do, quitting is a sensible strategy. For information about herbs that can help you stop smoking, see my book, *Herbs to Help You Breathe Freely.*

Physicians who study food sensitivities say the most common offenders are the foods we eat most often, such as wheat and milk, for, according to their theory, the body builds up an intolerance for them. Jean Carper listed the 20 foods most likely to aggravate rheumatoid arthritis as corn, wheat, bacon/pork, oranges, milk, oats, rye, eggs, beef, coffee, malt, cheese, grapefruit, tomato, peanuts, cane sugar, butter, lamb, lemon and soy. According to British authority L. Gail Darlington, corn and wheat are the worst offenders, triggering symptoms in more than half of the patients tested.

According to Jonathan Wright, M.D., a common denominator linking lupus, ulcerative colitis, Grave's disease, juvenile diabetes, vitiligo and other autoimmune diseases is a shared tissue type that is also common to those who have celiac disease (sprue). These illnesses may share an allergic reaction to the gluten and gliadin found in wheat, oats, barley, rye and other grains, though not corn or rice. Wright's lupus patients improved after eliminating most grains and all dairy products from their diets.

According to Sobel and Klein, authors of *Arthritis: What Works*, the most common offenders in rheumatoid and osteoarthritis are beef and other red meats, sugar and other sweets, fat and fried foods, refined table salt, caffeine, dairy products, nightshade vegetables, smoked or processed meats, pork, alcohol, junk food, refined starches such as white flour, additives, preservatives, acid foods, chocolate and—especially for gout patients—purines, which are substances that break down into uric acid in the body. Purines are found in organ meats, beef and other meats, mussels and other shellfish, herring, sardines, mackerel, fish roe and anchovies, all of which should be avoided by the gout patient. It is ironic that these same fatty cold-water fish bring relief to other forms of arthritis.

Research on the food-arthritis connection is still an open field, and every expert seems to have a different list of "most offending" foods. The lists are more than confusing; they are sometimes contradictory and always overwhelming, for they seem to contain every food most people eat every day. Restrictive diets are never easy, especially when they deviate from the social norm. Experimenting to find the foods your body reacts to takes time and effort, but freedom from pain and inflammation is a powerful incentive.

To test for food sensitivities and to overcome digestive problems that may be linked to arthritis, rheumatism and other inflammatory illnesses, see my book *Herbs to Improve Digestion*

THE RAW AND THE COOKED

Just as vegetarians consider arthritis a meat-eater's illness, raw-food enthusiasts call it a cooked-food disease. Experiments with the healing effects of raw food are practically unknown in the United States, but the biological clinics of Europe have repeatedly shown that raw foods cure disease. In Scandinavia, Switzerland, Germany, Austria and other countries, physicians treat cancer and every other illness, including arthritis and rheumatism, with raw foods, herbs and other natural therapies. Reports of their success and of related laboratory research and clinical trials are widely published in medical and scientific journals.

SPECIAL DIETS FOR ARTHRITIS

In addition to raw-food regimens, several special diets have been created for the treatment of arthritis, rheumatism and related illnesses. Most have other applications as well, but their effectiveness in the treatment of inflammatory diseases is well documented.

In the 1920s and '30s, Max Gerson, M.D., practiced medicine in Germany, where his specialty was diseases of the nervous system. After a natural foods diet cured his migraine headaches, he used the same therapy on patients. Even a case of lupus (cutaneous lupus erythematosus, or skin tuberculosis), which conventional medicine considers incurable, improved. Gerson's treatment of other lupus patients was equally successful, as were his cures of tuberculosis, meningitis, diabetes, cancer, arthritis, rheumatism and other chronic illnesses. In the late 1930s, Gerson left Nazi Germany for the United States, where he refined his program. It consisted of raw fruits and vegetables, freshly prepared juices, raw milk dishes, raw egg yolks, coffee enemas and glandular supplements such as raw liver extract. His success rate in curing cancer was dramatic, yet the medical establishment in the U.S. blocked the publication of his well-documented research and worked to revoke his license for practicing "unorthodox medicine."

Today the Gerson Institute, run by Charlotte Gerson, the doctor's daughter, specializes in curing "incurables" who have cancer, heart disease, diabetes, allergies, arthritis, rheumatism, asthma, hepatitis, lupus, multiple sclerosis, chronic fatigue syndrome and other illnesses. Workshops and lectures are given throughout the U.S., Canada and other countries.

Another nutritional approach to cancer, the Breuss Cancer Cure, has successfully treated arthritis, rheumatism, gout and other inflammatory illnesses. Developed in Germany by Rudolf Breuss and offered by clinics in Germany, Austria, Switzerland, Canada and other countries, the cancer program is a 42-day juice fast in which the only foods are freshly made raw juices, plain water and herb teas. For arthritis, degenerative joint inflammation, hip-joint arthritis, osteoporosis, ankylosing spondylitis and related illnesses, Breuss recommended 21 days of therapy, including frequent baths containing herbal teas such as horsetail, hay flower and oatstraw.

James K. Van Fleet, D.C., has devoted most of his career to the treatment of arthritis, rheumatism and related inflammatory illnesses. His approach, which has helped thousands, involves taking 1 tablespoon of peanut oil in juice every morning, plus a daily massage of affected areas with peanut oil (in case of an allergy to peanuts, substitute another oil); 1 tablespoon cod liver oil in juice at night; 1,500 or more mg of calcium and half as much magnesium daily; several alfalfa tablets and 3 to 4 cups of alfalfa tea daily; and ½ pound of cherries every day. In addition, eat mostly fresh fruits and vegetables, eat as much raw food as possible, drink 6 or more glasses of plain water daily, take appropriate vitamins and minerals, avoid packaged and processed foods, eliminate refined white sugar and fatty foods, avoid nightshades, reduce stress, laugh every day, exercise daily but with care, and be patient. In most cases, the author says, you will need a month of treatment for every year you have had the condition before its cure is complete.

Carlson Wade advocated "biological washing" for arthritis in his best-selling book *Inner Cleansing: How to Free Yourself from Joint-Muscle-Artery-*

Circulation Sludge. Wade blamed toxic wastes or free radicals for arthritis, rheumatism and other types of inflammation. To treat it, he recommended eating only raw foods and drinking fresh, raw juices for two days every week. For difficult or unresponsive cases, avoid nightshades as well. In addition, take cod liver oil and several times a week eat fish rich in omega-3 fatty acids: haddock, cod, pollack, sole, tuna, red snapper, flounder, turbot, rockfish, striped bass, ocean perch, whiting, carp, salmon, whitefish, herring and sablefish. Garlic is another part of the therapy, preferably three cloves daily. Last, he advocated hydrotherapy, a 15- to 20-minute bath in water slightly above body temperature followed by a hot 5-minute shower.

In the U.S., the process of elimination is seldom discussed in polite circles, television commercials for laxatives notwithstanding. Intestinal cleansing is an important part of many nutritional therapies, and a common side effect of many herbal detoxification programs is improvement in arthritis, rheumatism, gout, neuritis and other inflammatory illnesses.

THE IMPORTANCE OF JUICING

While it's true that Americans don't eat enough fiber, an impaired digestive tract may not be able to cope with a sudden supply of raw produce. Juicing is a popular therapy because juices are concentrated, nutritious and easy to assimilate. They are, in a sense, predigested. Someone whose stomach and intestines would be overwhelmed by even a few raw carrots can absorb the nutrients in five pounds of carrots just by swallowing their juice. Fresh juices contain all of the enzymes and nutrients found in the fruits or vegetables that made them.

Juicing is of special interest to arthritis patients because so many patients who go on a juice fast lasting several days experience complete relief from symptoms.

Some juice enthusiasts promote their machines and books on television, and most department stores and supermarkets stock electric juicers. If you're serious about juicing, it will be worth your while to invest in the best juicer you can afford. In addition to transforming fresh fruits and vegetables, these appliances can juice fresh herbs, making them easier to assimilate. Herbs such as parsley and fruits such as cherries play an important role in antiarthritis therapies.

Once you have a juicer and a good supply of produce, preferably organically grown, you can experiment with juice fasting—not true fasting, but going without solid food while drinking only juice and water or tea for several days or weeks—and other juice therapies. Juice fasting is a popular way to treat arthritis and similar disorders because it lets overworked organs rest while improving the body's absorption of nutrients. A gradual return to solid food and appropriate menu planning complete the cure.

Looking for a juice that treats inflammation? Here are suggestions from John Lust from his book *Drink Your Troubles Away*.

For arthritis, drink the following juice combinations:
1. Carrot 8 ounces, celery 8 ounces.
2. Carrot 6 ounces, beet 5 ounces, cucumber 5 ounces.
3. During acute stages, drink 1 pint to 1 quart celery juice daily.

For gout:
1. Carrot 8 ounces, celery 4 ounces, spinach 2 ounces, parsley 2 ounces.
2. Carrot 8 ounces, spinach 8 ounces.
3. Carrot 6 ounces, beet 5 ounces, cucumber 5 ounces.
4. Carrot 8 ounces, beet 4 ounces, coconut 4 ounces.

For rheumatism:
1. Juice of ½ lemon in a glass of warm water in the morning, then: Carrot 8 ounces, celery 8 ounces.
2. Carrot 8 ounces, orange 8 ounces.
3. Carrot 12 ounces, spinach 4 ounces.
4. Carrot 6 ounces, beet 5 ounces, cucumber 5 ounces.
5. Carrot 6 ounces, beet 5 ounces, celery 5 ounces.

SPROUTING HERBS AND SEEDS FOR LIVE FOODS

One of the easiest ways to obtain fresh, live, organically grown food is to sprout it yourself. Among the foods emphasized in livefood programs are wheat grass, barley grass and other tray-grown greens, as well as sprouts grown in jars or baskets.

Wheat grass is rich in vitamins A, C and E and it

contains all of the known minerals and trace elements, especially calcium, phosphorus, iron, potassium, sulphur, sodium, cobalt and zinc. These nutrients are stored in the seed; they don't result from anything in the soil, although adding liquid trace minerals or seaweed extract to the soaking water boosts the mineral content of whatever you grow. Recent research indicates that grasses are high in B vitamins and they contain approximately 70 percent chlorophyll, one of nature's greatest healers. Chlorophyll helps eliminate toxins from the body, purify the liver, clean the bloodstream, improve digestion and balance blood sugar. Because it loses nutrients quickly, wheat grass juice should be used within 10 minutes of pressing. Cut grass can be refrigerated in sealed plastic bags for up to a week. Frozen wheat grass juice keeps for several weeks, although it is not as effective as freshly pressed juice.

NUTRITIONAL SUPPLEMENTS

Research has shown that certain nutrients can help relieve inflammation. Medical journals published in the U.S. and other countries have documented the effectiveness of large quantities of vitamin C as well as smaller amounts of vitamins A, B1, B6, B12, E and niacinamide, a form of vitamin B3 that improves joint flexibility, in treating and preventing arthritis. Vitamin B6 may be a key nutrient for rheumatoid arthritis and it helps heal Heberden's nodes, an osteoarthritic condition in which bony lumps form at finger joints, as well as carpal tunnel syndrome. Karl Folkers, Ph.D., discovered that patients with carpal tunnel syndrome actually had a severe vitamin B6 deficiency, and vitamin B6 supplements (pyridoxine) made such an improvement that they didn't require orthopedic hand surgery. Even patients who had significant symptoms for 10 to 15 years showed improvement.

Aspirin destroys vitamin C, so vitamin C depletion is common in arthritis patients, as are low zinc and folic acid levels, which may also be drug-related. In the treatment of acute arthritis, such as that caused by advanced Lyme disease, Michael Murray, N.D., recommends 3 to 6 grams of vitamin C daily, taken in divided doses. Smaller amounts may be helpful for milder inflammation. Vitamin C's proponents use bowel tolerance as a guideline: when the body has absorbed all the vitamin C it can use, mild diarrhea develops.

Iron is one mineral that should not be taken in supplement form by arthritics because large amounts are suspected of contributing to pain, swelling and joint destruction. To prevent an iron deficiency, use blackstrap molasses as a sweetener and eat foods that are rich in iron, such as broccoli and cauliflower.

According to Julian Whitaker, M.D., the supplement glucosamine sulfate can be very effective not only in treating but also in reversing arthritis because it stimulates the production of connective tissue and new cartilage growth.

Calcium has a special place in the treatment of arthritis. Essential for bone, joint, muscle and ligament health, calcium works best in combination with magnesium. Not only do most Americans consume too little magnesium, their high protein diets contain excessive phosphorus, which binds magnesium, making it unavailable to the body, and excessive protein causes the body to excrete calcium.

Carl J. Reich, M.D., is best known for his work with calcium and vitamin D, which is necessary for calcium's assimilation. For over 30 years, Reich treated thousands of patients with a combination of vitamin D, calcium and magnesium. Not only did this therapy help prevent osteoporosis, it improved the condition of patients with rheumatoid arthritis, osteoarthritis and asthma in 60 to 90 percent of cases.

Because arthritis, bursitis and bone spurs involve calcium deposits, calcium is sometimes blamed for these conditions, just as it used to be blamed for kidney stones. According to Joel Wallach, N.D., calcium deposits are caused not by excess calcium in the diet but by its opposite, a calcium deficiency. Medical studies show that people with the highest calcium intake have the lowest incidence of kidney stones.

Boron has received attention from medical researchers in recent years for its ability to prevent calcium loss. Apples, pears, grapes and other fruits are rich sources of boron, and so are nuts and green vegetables.

Shark cartilage has become famous for its ability

to reduce inflammation and other symptoms of arthritis. Clinical trials show that oral shark cartilage supplements taken before meals are effective in over half the patients tested after less than three weeks in some cases. Medical studies have demonstrated shark cartilage's benefits in the treatment of cancer, eye diseases, lupus, inflammatory bowel disease, scleroderma, yeast infections and skin diseases. The supplement is not recommended for pregnant women or those with heart disease or liver dysfunction, and large amounts of the powder or capsules can cause gastric upset.

Sharks aren't the only source of cartilage. Bovine trachea cartilage is also receiving attention for its ability to reduce inflammation. This substance is rich in chondroitin sulfate, a natural joint lubricant and anti-inflammatory agent that has been shown to stimulate regeneration of damaged cartilage tissues and improve synovial fluid viscosity. Bovine trachea cartilage and purified chondroitin sulfate supplements are sold for human use, but their most enthusiastic users may be veterinarians, horse owners and people with dogs and cats. Arthritis, knee lameness, bone spurs, painful hocks, swelling and pain have all improved with their use.

Australia's sea cucumber is another friend of arthritics. Sea cucumbers, which are animals, not vegetables, emit defensive toxins that have an anti-inflammatory effect when taken orally. Rheumatoid arthritis, osteoarthritis, tendinitis, sports injuries and related conditions often respond well; in fact, research at the University of Queensland in 1992 found that sea cucumber is not only anti-inflammatory but antiarthritic, treating the disease as well as its symptoms. Australia's Department of Health has approved sea cucumber as an effective treatment for arthritis, and researchers such as Mitchell Kurk, M.D., director of the Biomedical Revitalization Center of Lawrence, N.Y., have found that approximately 70 percent of the arthritis patients they treat with the product improve.

Because heat destroys the enzymes in food, some arthritis researchers theorize that inflammatory conditions may improve if patients add digestive enzymes to their food whenever they eat something cooked, baked, fried, steamed or boiled. Lina Lee, Ph.D., advises patients to take the plant enzymes protease, analase, lipase and cellulase to increase digestion. This is a simple strategy because digestive enzymes are inexpensive, widely sold and safe.

The digestive enzyme bromelain, which comes from pineapples, has been the subject of numerous studies. According to the *Textbook of Natural Medicine*, it is effective in virtually all inflammatory conditions, regardless of cause. It works by blocking the formation of certain prostaglandins (hormone-like substances) that trigger inflammation while increasing the body's levels of natural anti-inflammatory substances and breaking up fibrin, a substance that collects in areas of inflammation, leading to pain and swelling.

Intestinal bacteria are important for many digestive functions, and an abundance of "friendly" bacteria, such as *Lactobacillus acidophilus* and *Bifidus* bacteria, provide important nutritional support for everyone, especially those who have taken antibiotics. No matter what your state of health, you can probably improve it by taking acidophilus/bifidus bacteria supplements. Because arthritis is so closely linked to diet, nutrition and digestion, it makes sense to improve the body's assimilation of nutrients by adding friendly bacteria to the daily diet.

In addition to increasing the population of friendly bacteria in their digestive tracts, many arthritics can relieve their symptoms and improve their digestion with hydrochloric acid, or HCl. We are so conditioned by the advertising campaigns of antacid products that most Americans assume their indigestion is caused by too much, not too little, HCl, but medical research indicates that 10 to 15 percent of the general population has this problem. Among those in poor health, the percentage is higher, and an estimated 50 percent of those over age 60 have insufficient hydrochloric acid.

Many illnesses are associated with low stomach acidity, including osteoporosis, rheumatoid arthritis and lupus erythematosus.

Alternative Therapies for Arthritis and Inflammatory Diseases

ENVIRONMENTAL ALLERGIES

Can arthritis and other rheumatic illnesses be caused by environmental allergies? The first physician to suggest a connection was Theron Randolph, M.D., the founder of environmental medicine. After testing over a thousand arthritics, Randolf found significant links between their arthritis and their reactions to foods, chemicals, perfumes, tobacco and other substances. According to Marshall Mandell, M.D., former director of the New England Foundation for Allergic and Environmental Diseases, "Allergies may or may not cause arthritis, but they definitely play a major role in a majority of cases because they often aggravate and perpetuate the condition." When allergenic substances are eliminated, avoided or contacted less frequently, the arthritis is usually relieved or eliminated. In tests of over 6,000 patients, Mandell found that foods, chemicals, grasses, pollen, molds and other airborne substances caused allergic reactions in the joints of nearly 85 percent of the arthritics he tested. Other studies have shown that food additives, bacteria, yeasts, fungi and protozoa can trigger or aggravate arthritic symptoms.

One way to identify possible allergens is to isolate the patient in a "clean" (allergy-free) environment for five days during which the patient consumes nothing but untreated, uncontaminated spring water. Foods and chemicals are introduced one at a time, and the patient's reaction is carefully monitored. Knowing what chemicals or conditions to avoid has lessened the arthritic symptoms of many who have undergone this analysis.

YOU AREN'T ILL, YOU'RE JUST DEHYDRATED

Unique among alternative therapists is F. Batmanghelidj, M.D., author of *Your Body's Many Cries for Water.* Dr. Batmanghelidj's basic premise, which has been endorsed by reputable physicians, scientists and researchers worldwide, is that many illnesses, including arthritis and rheumatism, are caused by dehydration. His treatment could not be simpler: Drink more water. When the body is fully hydrated, cartilage is properly lubricated and fluids circulate through joint cavities as joints are moved. When there is insufficient fluid, inflammation results.

In addition to three or more quarts of plain drinking water every day (juices, coffee, tea and other beverages don't count), Batmanghelidj recommended small amounts of salt. In fact, he wrote that in arthritis, salt shortage is often a contributing factor.

According to Batmanghelidj, pain and local swelling of joint surfaces often disappear after sufficient water and salt are consumed and, more important, the joint structure begins to repair itself.

For a complete description of Dr. Batmanghelidj's therapies, see his books *How to Deal with Back Pain and Rheumatoid Joint Pain* and *Your Body's Many Cries for Water.*

SALT BATHS

Along with hot baths, cold showers, ice packs and heat treatments, salt scrubs are a standard spa therapy for arthritis. Salt stimulates the skin, increases circulation, removes dead cells and increases nerve activity. Add just enough water to make a thick paste, then dampen your body with a sponge, scoop up a handful and rub as briskly as you can without irritating the skin, massaging feet, ankles, knees, hands, arms, back, chest and abdomen. Fill the tub with warm water and relax, rinsing the salt off. For an invigorating skin-softening treatment, mix salt with massage oil instead of water and proceed as above. The oil will be slippery, so place a towel under your feet before standing.

For a luxurious salt bath, use enough unrefined sea salt to make the water ocean-salty and stay in the tub as long as possible. Ocean water's healing properties have made seaside health spas popular throughout Europe, especially on the coast of France.

BEE STINGS AND OTHER VENOMS

Among the more colorful—and painful—treatments for inflammatory disorders is apitherapy, or the use of bee stings. In the July 1995 edition of *Natural Health*, Andrew Weil answered a reader's question by writing:

> Bee-venom therapy has a long history of use for alleviation of rheumatoid arthritis and some other auto-immune and inflammatory disorders, including multiple sclerosis. Although the procedure is safe, most doctors, knowing nothing about it, warn people away from it. Beekeepers are much more knowledgeable and are usually the best source of information on the subject.

Although purified honey bee venom is available for injection, most apitherapists say it is better and more convenient to apply the bees with tweezers. Dosages range from a cautious one or two stings every other day to 50 or 60 stings per day. Mild forms of inflammation often respond after just a few stings, while more serious conditions, such as osteoarthritis and rheumatoid arthritis, may require weeks or months of regular stings.

According to veteran apitherapist and beekeeper Charles Mraz of Middlebury, Vermont, about 80 percent of the thousands of people he has treated in the past 60 years have either fully recovered from their ailments or significantly improved. More than 1,500 papers on the medical benefits of bee venom have been published in European and Asian scientific journals, and though few American researchers have experimented with the procedure, scientists at Walter Reed Medical Hospital have injected bee venom into arthritic dogs with consistently positive results.

An estimated 2 percent of the population is allergic to bee venom, and for these people, apitherapy is, of course, not recommended. Anyone considering the therapy should be tested for potential allergic reactions.

Herbs for Arthritis

The following herbs are just a few of the hundreds prescribed around the world for inflammation. All are sold in U.S. health food stores and herb shops, most in a variety of products, including teas, liquid extracts, tinctures (alcohol extracts), capsules, tablets and powders.

To make your own herbal preparations, buy herbs from a reputable dealer and, if possible, purchase organically grown or wildcrafted herbs that have been carefully dried at low temperatures and stored away from heat, light and humidity. If you enjoy gardening and outdoor activities, grow the plants yourself or gather them in the wild from safe, unpolluted sources. Take an herb class or study field guides, herb books and the catalogs of mail order herb nurseries for information on growing, gathering and storing your harvest.

HERBAL PREPARATIONS

Tea Brewing

To brew an *infusion* (recommended for most leaves and blossoms), pour boiling water over loose tea in a jar or teapot, cover and let stand for 10 to 15 minutes. Strain and serve. To brew a *decoction* (recommended for most bark and roots), place the herb in a covered pot with water, bring just to a boil, reduce heat and simmer for 10 to 15 minutes. Remove from heat, let stand an additional 5 minutes. Strain and serve. To brew a beverage-strength tea, use about 1 teaspoon dried herb per cup of water; to brew a medicinal strength tea, use 2 teaspoons to 1 tablespoon dried herb per cup of water. Double or triple these quantities for fresh herbs. For convenience, brew 4 cups (1 quart) tea at a time. A pot or jar of tea brewed late in the day can be left overnight before straining; in fact, overnight brewing is recommended by many herbalists, especially for medicinal teas. Most teas can be kept at room temperature for one day or refrigerated for several days without spoiling.

Because medicinal teas often have a bitter, unpleasant taste, especially for the American palate, which has been trained to prefer sweet and salty flavors, many people sweeten their teas with sugar, honey or concentrated flavors. While nutritionists who study arthritis frown on the use of sugar and honey, they do approve blackstrap molasses because of its iron content, important to arthritics who are warned not to take iron supplements. For calorie-free sweetening, the recommended herb is stevia, a plant that thrives in desert climates and which is used around the world as a sugar substitute. Stevia does not taste exactly like sugar, but a pinch can give a pleasantly sweet taste to any tea. For several years stevia was hard to find in U.S. herb shops because of an FDA embargo imposed after lobbying efforts by the manufacturers of artificial sweeteners. Today it is available without restriction. A dash of apple juice also works well as a sweetener.

External Applications

Any discussion of herbal teas would be incomplete without a brief discussion of their external applications.

A *poultice* is a wet herbal pack applied directly to an inflamed, irritated, swollen, infected or injured part of the body. While poultices can be made of fresh mashed herbs, they can also be made of the residue left after brewing tea.

Poultices are usually applied cool rather than hot. Some herbalists recommend spreading a thin layer of olive oil or castor oil before applying the plant material. Use whatever will hold the poultice in place for several hours: bandages, plastic wrap, cheesecloth, muslin, etc. A layer of plastic over the poultice helps prevent fabric stains.

A *compress* is an application of cold herbal tea on a saturated towel, diaper or thick cloth. Use medicinal-strength infusions or decoctions for this purpose. To treat a painful bruise or to relieve inflammation in a joint that feels hot or swollen, chill a strong **peppermint** tea, then soak the cloth and wring it just until it stops dripping. The compress should be wet enough to stay cold for several minutes. When it warms to body temperature, soak it again, adding ice as needed to keep the tea cold. Repeat until the treatment has lasted 15 to 20 minutes. Dry the skin gently.

A *fomentation* is a hot compress. Fomentations increase circulation and soothe injuries. They often bring relief to painful joints, although it's worth experimenting with both cold compresses and hot fomentations to discover which provides the most relief. Wearing rubber gloves, saturate a thick cloth with strong, hot, strained tea, wring it gently, then unfold it to let it cool slightly. You don't want it to burn or scald, but for best results it must be as hot as possible. Test the temperature against your inner arm. When it's hot but not too hot, apply it to the desired area and cover with a thick folded towel to retain heat. Repeat after 10 minutes.

Hydrotherapy is a healing art in itself. A quart of strong **oatstraw, peppermint, chamomile, comfrey, lavender, ginger, lemon balm** or **sweet spice** tea added to your bath is both an herbal and aromatherapy treatment. An effective therapy for muscle soreness and arthritis is to add salts as well as herbal teas to your bath. For a luxurious spa treatment, look for bath salts from the Dead Sea or add a little seaweed to your salt bath. Try combining any quantity of table or sea salt, epsom salts (magnesium sulfate) from the drug store or supermarket, baking soda (sodium bicarbonate) and borax, the laundry product. Dissolve at least four cups of this blend in hot water as you fill the tub. Adjust the temperature so it's comfortably warm; then, just before you climb in, add your quart of herbal tea.

Few remedies are as soothing to aching bones and sore joints as **mustard** baths, which are also recommended for winter colds. For a hydrotherapy treat, combine Epsom salts, sea salt, borax and/or baking soda in any proportions to make a basic bath salt. In a gallon-sized Zip-lock plastic bag, combine 4 cups of the salt mixture with 1 cup powdered mustard. Knead the closed bag to distribute the mustard evenly and break up any lumps in the salt. Add several drops of **eucalyptus** essential oil or **tea tree oil** or add 4 tablespoons powdered ginger and mix well. Empty the bag under hot running water and fill the tub to a comfortably warm temperature. Soak for at least 15 to 20 minutes. For best results, pat yourself dry, wrap yourself in blankets (perspiration is desired) and stay warm for half an hour.

Foot baths, sitz baths and even hand baths continue the hydrotherapy theme. Some inflammatory conditions respond well to alternating immersions in hot and cold water, and this is true for fomentations and compresses as well as baths.

Capsules

Herbal tea companies often sell empty gelatin capsules and hand-operated capping devices to speed their filling. Herbs can be ground in any electric spice or coffee grinder. To fill your own capsules, which allows you to control the quality and proportion of ingredients, buy an inexpensive grinder and use it just for herbs. (Use a separate grinder for coffee.) Wear a pollen mask to avoid breathing herb dust and wipe the grinder clean after each use. Some herbs, such as cloves, contain essential oils that dissolve plastic parts if their residue is left in the grinder. Vegetarian capsules are available through health food stores and herb shops; regular gelatin capsules, which are less expensive, are made from animal parts. Note that certain aromatic spices (cloves again, and there may be others) cause vegetable gelatin caps to shatter after a day or two of storage, though they work perfectly well for all herbs and most spices.

Tinctures

To make a tincture, which is a concentrated medicinal extract, place a handful of fresh or dried herbs in a quart jar and cover them with 80-proof (or higher proof) vodka, rum, whisky or brandy until the alcohol covers the herbs by at least two inches. Alternatively, use vegetable glycerine instead of alcohol, or combine the two. Vegetable glycerine is a sweet thick fluid that extracts most but not all of the plant constituents dissolved by alcohol and is a popular ingredient in children's tinctures. Cider vinegar can be used to make tinctures, too, but it dissolves fewer plant compounds and has a shorter shelf life. Cider vinegar tinctures last a year or more when stored away from heat and light and even longer if refrigerated, and they can be used in salad dressings and other foods. Vegetable glycerine tinctures last longer and alcohol tinctures keep indefinitely.

Whatever liquid you use, cover the jar tightly, leave it in a warm place and shake it daily for at least two weeks, adding more alcohol, glycerine or vinegar as dry herbs absorb the liquid. The longer it steeps, the stronger the tincture. Strain and pour into storage bottles, an activity that many herbalists conduct at the full moon. For a double-strength tincture, let the tincture stand for one month, then pour the strained liquid over new herbs and repeat the process.

There is much confusion about tincture dosage, a misunderstanding that herbalist Rosemary Gladstar attributes to the caution of small companies marketing tinctures in the 1960s. "The only similar products were homeopathic preparations," she explains, "and their doses are measured in drops. Herbal tinctures are entirely different, and they should be taken by the half-teaspoon, teaspoon or tablespoon, not by the drop." Anyone buying, making or taking herbal tinctures should know that disappointing results may not be caused by a tincture's herbal ingredients but rather by doses that are entirely too small. Tinctures can be taken straight or diluted in tea, water or fruit juice. Some tinctures, such as **arnica** and **nettle,** have important external applications; they are used as liniments. While liniments can be made with isopropyl or rubbing alcohol, which is poisonous if swallowed, many herbalists prefer to use grain alcohol for this purpose.

Infused Oils

To make an infused oil for external application, as in a rub or salve, start with dry or partly dry herbs. If you are using fresh herbs, let them wilt because the high water content of freshly picked herbs may cause spoilage. Loosely fill a glass jar with herbs (leave extra room for expansion if the herbs are dry) and cover with the oil of your choice. Most herbalists recommend olive oil, but you can use peanut oil or any cold-pressed oil with good results, or blend several oils together. Health food stores carry almond, avocado, castor, coconut, jojoba, olive, corn, peanut, peach kernel, apricot kernel, grape seed, safflower, sesame, soybean, wheat germ, borage, evening primrose, rose hip and walnut oils as well as karite butter (shea butter or African nut butter), lanolin, cocoa butter and lecithin, all of which are appropriate ingredients. Because castor oil is viscous and sticky, it should be blended with other, more "slippery" oils, and because of their expense, evening primrose, rose hip, borage and vitamin E oils are usually added in small quantities.

Use a single or blended oil to cover the herbs and fill the jar almost to the top. For best results and to prevent rancidity, use a canning jar or any jar you can seal tightly and clean the jar rim and lid to remove any trace of oil. Screw the lid on tight to prevent any leakage or air exchange. Leave the jar in a warm place, preferably in full sunlight, for several weeks, inverting the jar every few days. Alternatively, place the jar on a small rack in a large pot of water and let the water simmer for several hours. Or simply place the herbs and oil in the top of a double boiler and, with cover in place, heat the oil over simmering water for an hour or more.

Appropriate herbs for arthritis massage oils and rubbing salves include **comfrey** leaf or root, **arnica** blossoms, **boswella**, **calendula** blossoms, **St. John's wort** blossoms, **chamomile** blossoms, **devil's claw**, **feverfew**, **meadowsweet** and **white willow**. For warmth, add powdered **mustard**, freshly ground **cloves**, **cinnamon**, **ginger** and/or **cayenne pepper** (experiment cautiously with cayenne if you believe you are nightshade-sensitive; test a small amount on a small area first). For pain relief, add essential oil of **wintergreen** and/or **peppermint**. Start with small batches and experiment, keeping track of ingredients and quantities until you find a combination you like. Add several drops of a favorite essential oil for fragrance, as desired. The essential oils of clove, **cinnamon** and other sweet spices have a warming influence and pleasant fragrance, but be sure to dilute them in oil before applying to the skin or bath water. Small amounts of cinnamon oil can actually burn the skin.

HERBAL CATEGORIES

Herbs are defined according to their therapeutic benefits, and you will find the following terms used in herbal reference books. The categories of interest in the treatment of arthritis and related illnesses are alternatives, analgesics, anti-inflammatories, antirheumatics, antispasmodics, circulatory stimulants, nervines, rubefacients and sedatives.

ALTERATIVE herbs, traditionally known as blood purifiers, gradually improve the body's overall condition by enhancing digestion and the assimilation of nutrients while eliminating toxins and neutralizing acidic conditions. Generally high in vitamins, minerals and other nutrients, they have a tonic influence—that is, they restore and strengthen the entire system rather than any specific part. The alteratives most useful in the treatment of inflammation include **bog bean**, **devil's claw**, **nettle** and **sarsaparilla**.

An ANALGESIC is any substance that relieves pain. Most analgesic herbs reduce pain signals to the brain, easing discomfort, but like aspirin and other pharmaceutical analgesics, they do not affect the illness itself. **Skullcap**, **chamomile** and **valerian** are examples.

An ANTI-INFLAMMATORY herb does just what its name implies: it reduces inflammation. Some herbs contain salicylates, so they act like aspirin (**willow bark** and **meadowsweet**, for example) and others help eliminate the cause of inflammation, reducing or stopping the disease's progress (**feverfew, boswella**).

ANTIRHEUMATIC herbs are not so much specifics for rheumatism as they are alternatives that gradually correct imbalances in the body, repairing an unhealthy state to a healthy one. They work gradually to correct the underlying cause of rheumatic disease and can be taken daily for long periods (**alfalfa, bog bean, celery seed, sarsaparilla, feverfew**).

An ANTISPASMODIC relieves or prevents involuntary muscle spasms or cramps and helps lessen the impact of friction on the joints (**black cohosh, cramp bark**).

CIRCULATORY STIMULANTS activate and increase circulation and digestion, increasing the flow of blood through the tissues around joints and enhancing the effectiveness of other herbs taken at the same time (**prickly ash, cayenne, ginger**).

NERVINES are herbs that calm and soothe the nerves, reducing stress, tension and anxiety. They strengthen, tone, calm and nourish the nervous system (**black cohosh, valerian, skullcap, oatstraw, chamomile**) and are used as supporting or secondary herbs in arthritis formulas.

A RUBEFACIENT, applied externally, stimulates capillary dilation and causes skin redness by drawing blood to the area, relieving inflammation and congestion; herbs in this category have a warming effect (**cayenne, ginger, cloves, mustard**) and are used in sports rubs, liniments and therapeutic massage oils.

SEDATIVE herbs reduce anxiety, slow the pulse and other body functions, relieve stress and promote tranquility. They do not have the same effects as tranquilizing drugs; their influence is gentler and more subtle, and they have no adverse side effects. For those with rheumatoid arthritis, which has strong psychological connections, sedative nervines help prevent the flare-ups that often accompany stress; for anyone in pain, they help ensure a good night's sleep, which is vital to healing. Examples include **valerian, passionflower, black cohosh, chamomile** and **skullcap**.

Some of the following herbs have been tested in clinical trials or animal experiments, and all have a long history of clinical use in the treatment of rheumatoid arthritis, osteoarthritis, gout, ankylosing spondylitis, carpal tunnel syndrome, bursitis, neuritis, neuralgia, bone spurs, sciatica or related conditions. In general, if an herb works for one of these disorders, it will work for others. Every human body is different, and it is safe to assume that no one will find all of them effective or that any single herb will be effective for everyone. These herbs are sold by themselves and in blends of different kinds. In general, herbalists suggest that you give an herb a trial period of up to three months or even more before deciding that it doesn't work. Of course, if you have an adverse or allergic reaction to any herb, discontinue use.

ALFALFA *(Medicago sativa)*

Alfalfa has been used for centuries to treat arthritis, gout, rheumatism and related illnesses. Containing up to 50 percent protein and an abundance of beta-carotene, chlorophyll, octacosanol, saponins, sterols, flavonoids, vitamins, amino acids, minerals, trace elements and other nutrients, alfalfa has a long-standing reputation as a highly nutritious, appetite-stimulating herb for vitality. Ancient Arabs were the first to document its nutritional benefits, and they gave alfalfa its name, which means "father of all foods."

Alfalfa is often called an herbal tonic, which means that it restores and strengthens the entire system, not just specific organs or parts of the body. Because of its high nutrient value and its ability to affect lipid metabolism and plant steroids, an estimated 10 to 20 percent of those who take alfalfa tea, capsules, tablets, tinctures or powders experience a significant reduction in painful symptoms within weeks, and a higher percentage experience partial relief. Alfalfa is considered safe and is recommended for long-term use. Alfalfa supplements are also often used in the herbal treatment of arthritis in dogs and other pets, frequently with impressive results. However, raw alfalfa sprouts, widely sold in markets and health food stores, are not recommended for rheumatic conditions.

ALOE VERA (*Aloe vera*)

Once exotic, aloe vera has become ubiquitous. The spiny succulent is a popular house plant, and its healing gel is a highly praised treatment for burns, sunburn, abrasions, cuts, wounds, scrapes and insect bites. Aloe vera juice is a popular liquid supplement, and capsules are available as well. Used internally, aloe vera can have a harsh laxative effect unless the bitter rind is removed; the slippery gel from inside the leaf is not cathartic.

Some have promoted aloe vera as a cure-all, claiming spectacular results in almost every illness, including arthritis. Because there are many aloe preparations made by different manufacturing processes, some diluted and others concentrated, the marketplace can be confusing. But whether they apply it as a lotion or take it internally, thousands of users claim it has brought them relief from arthritis. In the *Aloe Vera Handbook*, Max B. Skousen wrote, "Most people who report some relief from arthritic symptoms say they drink one or two tablespoons at a time, two to four times a day, in juice or water." Although some reported immediate relief, most experienced improvement within two months.

ARNICA (*Arnica montana*)

Arnica is a small alpine plant with yellow blossoms. The flower heads, made into tea, tincture or massage oil, are anti-inflammatory and relieve the pain of bruises, sprains, rheumatism and inflammation. In *Medicinal Plants of the Pacific West*, Michael Moore wrote:

The primary uses for arnica have remained unchanged for centuries. The tincture, oil, salve, tea, or bruised fresh plant is used externally for bruises, hyperextensions, arthritis, bursitis, and myalgia. Arnica works by stimulating and dilating blood vessels. Good, diffused blood transport and circulation into injured, bruised, or inflamed tissues helps speed up resolution and removal of waste products. Arnica does not have the anesthesia of menthol or wintergreen or the counterirritation property of other aromatic balms, and should not be expected to have their immediate effects. Instead, in a few hours or overnight, it aids in removing the congestion that results from a bruise, sprain or hyperextension. In osteoarthritis, the stimulation supplied by arnica is a small but significant aid in increasing the absorption and drainage of the hyaline cartilage, lessening some of the early and chronic congestion of the joints that leads, gradually, to the overgrowth of bony cartilage characteristic of osteoarthritis. In rheumatoid arthritis, a highly variable condition with many elements of immunologic dysfunction, including overt autoimmunity, it is wise to try using arnica on the swollen joints for two or three days. If it helps the inflammation and shortens the length of morning stiffness in the primary joint, you will usually find that it can be used regularly without any problem. If it starts to overheat the joint or redden the skin below the surface, stop.

Arnica is not recommended for internal use.

BLACK COHOSH (*Cimicifuga racemosa*)

This antispasmodic, alternative and nervine herb is used in the treatment of rheumatic pains, rheumatoid arthritis, osteoarthritis, sciatica, neuralgia, neurological pain, muscle pain and sports injuries. The dried (not fresh) root and rhizome is brewed as a decoction by simmering 1 teaspoon root per cup of water.

BLUE-RED BERRIES

Cherries, hawthorn berries, blueberries, grapes and other dark red-blue berries are more properly a food than an herb, but they are so effective in the treatment of inflammatory illnesses, especially gout and arthritis, that they deserve consideration here. These berries are rich sources of compounds that improve collagen metabolism and reduce joint inflammation. The famous botanist Linnaeus reportedly cured his gout by eating large quantities of strawberries morning and night, which led him to call them a "blessing of the gods." More recently, a gout "strawberry cure" of eating nothing but strawberries for several days was made popular by the French herbalist Maurice Mésségué. James Van Fleet prescribes ½ cup of cherries daily for his arthritis patients, in keeping with that fruit's well-established reputation as a cure. During summer months, when these fruits are abundant, try to eat at least ½ cup daily, preferably more. If you drink fresh juices, add them to your juicer as often as possible. People have benefitted from canned, frozen, bottled, dried and even candied cherries, but for best results, make fresh fruit your first choice.

BOG BEAN OR BUCKBEAN
(*Menyanthes trifoliata*)

Although it is far more familiar to Europeans than Americans, this herb is worth the search because bog bean leaves are a specific for rheumatism, osteoarthritis and rheumatoid arthritis. As it has a mild laxative effect, this herb should not be used if diarrhea or irritable bowel syndrome is a problem. Bog bean is best known for its stimulation of digestive fluids and bile production; it improves digestion. In *An Elder's Herbal*, herbalist David Hoffmann recommends bog bean tea made with 1 or 2 teaspoons of herb per cup of water 3 times daily, or ¼ to ¾ teaspoon tincture 3 times daily.

BOSWELLA (*Boswella serratta*)

A large, branching tree native to India that produces a gummy resin, boswella has a long history of medicinal use in that country. Today, researchers and clinicians are proving that boswella is a potent anti-inflammatory herb that effectively shrinks inflamed tissue by improving circulation and increasing synovial fluid viscosity. In studies at the Government Medical College in Jammu, India, nearly 70 percent of arthritis patients tested experienced good to excellent results against stiffness and pain.

In the U.S., much of boswella's favorable publicity comes from veterinarians and pet owners, for it is used with much success on dogs, cats and horses. Boswella capsules and powders are sold for human and animal use; boswella creams help relieve pain and inflammation externally. Note that boswella does not appear to reverse or cure arthritis, for when pet owners run out of the herb, their animals regress quickly.

BUPLEURUM (*Bupleurum spp.*) or BEI CHAI HU

This Chinese herb has a long history of use in a variety of conditions, including liver disease and allergies. Its anti-inflammatory effects make it an effective treatment for arthritis and related illnesses, though it is better known for its sedative, relaxing properties, its reduction of sugar cravings and its use in the treatment of premenstrual symptoms and migraine headaches. Bupleurum strengthens the immune system and, because of its antibacterial and antiviral properties, can be taken to ward off colds and flu.

CAT'S CLAW (*Uncaria tomentosa*) or UNA DE GATO

In 1993, cat's claw was little known in America, but a year later it was making headlines and today this "wondrous new medicinal herb from Peru's Amazon rain forest" is recommended for nearly every illness known to pets and humans.

Cat's claw, known in Spanish as *Uña de Gato*, is a woody vine that grows over a hundred feet in length. Its sharp, curving thorns look just like a cat's claws. For centuries, native Indians have used the bark of the vine's root to prepare a medicinal decoction to treat tumors and other serious diseases.

Richard Gerber, M.D., believes that cat's claw shows "great promise for the treatment of arthritis when taken internally, either by making a tea or taking capsules of the herb. European research has found the herb has very low toxicity even in large amounts. It may be especially beneficial for individuals with painful joints, who cannot take conventional medicines because of stomach upset and other drug side effects."

Although cat's claw is available in capsules, that form may not be as effective as the tea. In addition to questioning the quality of cat's claw in capsules, the Austrian physician Klaus Keplinger, who has received patents for his cat's claw extracts, believes that the herb should never be taken raw, only cooked, which is its traditional method of preparation. Keplinger recommends making a decoction by cooking 20 grams cat's claw (0.7 ounce net weight, or about 1 cup shredded bark) in 1 quart water at 80 degrees Centigrade (176 degrees Fahrenheit, a slow simmer) for 45 minutes. Let cool 10 minutes, filter through paper and add enough water to make one full quart. Refrigerate. Mix 2 ounces tea with warm water and drink on an empty stomach once per day.

CAYENNE PEPPER (*Capsicum frutescens*)

Cayenne is the spice that gives chili its bite. An all-purpose stimulant, cayenne is a general tonic for the entire body and a specific for the circulatory and digestive systems. Because it's a member of the nightshade family, cayenne should not be taken by those who are sensitive to these plants, but those who don't have an adverse reaction to peppers can enjoy its fiery flavor or take it in capsules to improve circulation and mobility. Cayenne is an important ingredient in many sports rubs and massage creams. A rubefacient, cayenne increases the flow of blood to the skin and joints, and ointments containing it have a long history of use in treating lumbago and rheumatic pain. Use it in moderation because it can cause a burning sensation. However, this sensation decreases with frequent use.

CELERY SEED (*Apium graveolens*)

This familiar culinary spice can be brewed as a tea (infuse 2 teaspoons seed per cup of water) or made into a tincture for relief from inflammation and rheumatic symptoms. Celery seed has mild diuretic action and acts as a urinary antiseptic, and it has digestive benefits as well. Drink 1 cup of tea or ¼ to ½ teaspoon of tincture 3 times daily. Consider this a supporting herb in arthritis formulas.

CHAMOMILE (*Matricaria chamomilla*)

Chamomile, better known as a digestive tonic and sleep aid, plays a supportive role in the treatment of arthritis by making a soothing, relaxing tea that helps reduce inflammation, muscle spasms and anxiety. A cup of chamomile tea just before bed ensures a good night's sleep.

DEVIL'S CLAW ROOT (*Harpagophytum procumbens*)

Devil's claw has become, especially in Europe, a primary treatment for arthritis and rheumatism. Native to South Africa, devil's claw was tested in African and German hospitals and clinics after World War II. In 1958, the first published report of this research described its effectiveness in reducing inflammation and swelling in experimentally induced arthritis.

After the plant's active component, *harpagoside*, was identified, it was tested in rigorous pharmacological screening trials that validated its anti-inflammatory properties. Wholeroot preparations were found to be superior to pure harpagoside, and both were determined to be safe. In *Herbal Tonic Therapies*, Daniel B. Mowrey, Ph.D., reported:

> Recent studies have found that devil's claw preparations are generally well-suited for the treatment of chronic rheumatism, arthritis, gout, spondylosis-induced lower back pain, neuralgia, headaches and lumbago. One study found that its anti-inflammatory effects equaled those of pyrazolone derivatives and the commonly prescribed antiarthritic phenylbutazone. Relief of pain is probably a side benefit of reduced inflammation. Improved motility in the joints is often reported, as well as improved feelings of well-being. Currently, physicians in Europe are injecting devil's claw extract directly into arthritic joints, where it acts much like cortisone in terms of reducing inflammation. As is the case with most arthritis treatments, not everybody benefits, but there are enough who do to warrant further investigation of this plant and to recommend it as a possible treatment option.

The Canadian Bureau of Drug Research has shown that devil's claw has no known toxicity.

FEVERFEW (*Tanacetum parthenium*)

This is a bitter tasting green plant that blossoms with daisy-like white petals around a yellow center. Not quite pretty enough to be a cut flower and so unattractive to bees that it actually repels them, feverfew remained an obscure herb until its ability to prevent migraine headaches put it back into nurseries, seed catalogs, home gardens and health food stores around the world.

Much of the credit for feverfew's popularity belongs to Ken Hancock, a bus supervisor in England, who sent letters to newspaper editors asking for information about the herb when he learned it might help his wife's headaches. In time, he received hundreds of letters from around the world documenting users' experiences in their own words. Enough of the correspondence was published in newspapers to make feverfew a best-selling herb in England.

Hancock recounted the correspondence in his book, *Feverfew: Your Headache May Be Over.* Not only did feverfew prevent migraine headaches in most users, it also relived their arthritis, psoriasis, premenstrual and menopausal symptoms, insomnia, stress, and many other ailments.

Research proving feverfew's effectiveness in the treatment of migraines and arthritis has been reported in *The British Medical Journal* and *Lancet* since the 1970s. The herb's taste is so bitter that most people prefer taking capsules to eating the fresh plant or drinking its tea, and a few users experience mouth and throat irritation from an allergic reaction. No other adverse side effects have been documented, and long-term users have been monitored for blood pressure, liver function and other factors for several years. For best results, herbalist Christopher Hobbs recommends taking freeze-dried feverfew in capsules. Exposure to heat and improper drying destroy parthenolide, its active ingredient.

According to Hancock, onset-stage arthritis, monthly migraines, minor stress and insomnia should respond to a daily dosage of 125 mg dried herb. Arthritis accompanied by serious pain, stiffness and joint swelling, frequent migraines and ankylosing spondylitis usually respond to 125 mg given twice daily for 10 to 14 days; if relief is rapid, reduce the dosage to 125 mg once per day. Higher dosages may increase the chances of an allergic reaction.

For best results, take feverfew with food whenever possible; do not chew raw leaves if you grow the plant yourself (instead, swallow a 2 × 2.5-inch piece of leaf with food); if taking 250 mg daily, take half in the morning and half at night; do not take feverfew with high dosage blood pressure medication; avoid alcohol during the first two weeks of treatment (alcohol interferes with feverfew's effectiveness); and experiment to reduce the dosage when you begin to experience results.

Improvements caused by feverfew often continue for weeks, months and even years after treatment stops, suggesting that the herb actually helps cure the disease.

GINGER (*Zingiber officinale*)

This familiar cooking spice is a stimulant herb that enhances circulation and digestion. Ginger is so versatile that it is used for many conditions, and its ability to prevent nausea has made it a popular alternative to drugs that treat motion sickness and morning sickness. Applied externally, ginger increases circulation and brings warmth to painful joints. To make a warming ginger bath, grate fresh ginger root and place up to ¼ cup grated ginger (or substitute 2 tablespoons powdered ginger) in a cloth bag or washcloth; tie closed with yarn or string. Place the cloth under hot water as you fill the tub, then squeeze it from time to time to release more ginger, or apply the ginger cloth to sore joints. For an even more aromatic ginger bath, brew a strong ginger tea by simmering the fresh or dried ginger in 2 cups water for 5 minutes; let stand another 10 minutes, then strain into bath water. Fresh or powdered ginger can be added to any massage oil.

Dr. Krishna Srivastava, an internationally recognized medical researcher on spices at Odense University in Denmark, tested small daily doses of ginger on arthritis patients for three months, during which most experienced reduced pain, swelling and morning stiffness and increased mobility. One 50-year-old man began eating between one and two ounces of fresh ginger daily when he was diagnosed with rheumatoid arthritis. His symptoms diminished within one month; after three months he was completely free of pain, inflammation and swelling, and in the following ten years he experienced no recurrence of symptoms. Srivastava recommends that his arthritis patients take about 1 tablespoon fresh ginger or 500 mg (about ⅓ teaspoon) ground dried ginger three times daily. Ginger capsules are sold in health food stores.

HORSETAIL (*Equisetum arvense*)

Horsetail, a common weed in damp locations, plays a supportive role in the treatment of arthritis because of its high silicon content. Long a folk treatment for mending bones and connective tissue, horsetail's healing properties have been proven in clinical research. Horsetail stimulates the metabolic processes that repair bones and connective tissue, and its effectiveness in the treatment of arthritis and other inflammatory conditions may result from its ability to replace lost silicon in the body. Silicon levels decline with age, possibly due to a drop in hormone levels.

The famous Austrian herbalist Maria Treben recommended in *Health Through God's Pharmacy* that everyone over 40 drink a cup of horsetail infusion every day. "It helps stop the onset of gout, rheumatism and other similar complaints that tend to appear as one gets older," she wrote. "Make each cup last a whole day, taking little sips at regular intervals."

In addition to taking horsetail tea or capsules, traditional European arthritis treatments include horsetail baths. To make your own, simply brew a strong horsetail tea by covering ¼ cup dried horsetail with 1 quart boiling water in a glass jar, cover and let stand for half an hour. Strain into bath water.

MEADOWSWEET (*Filipendula ulmaria*)

Meadowsweet blossoms are used in many arthritis tea blends because of their antirheumatic, anti-inflammatory influence. In addition, the plant is a natural antacid that aids digestion, treats gastritis and peptic ulcers and increases the intestine's ability to absorb nutrients.

Meadowsweet's almond-scented flowers were used in the Middle Ages as a strewing herb. Walking on the plant released its fragrance and freshened the air. Meadowsweet contains salacin, a natural form of the key ingredient in aspirin. According to William Keller, Ph.D., "Once the salicin from meadowsweet is in the stomach, it breaks down to create salicylic acid, and basically that's what happens when you take an aspirin. It definitely has an analgesic effect."

Meadowsweet is often combined with white willow bark in equal proportions for improved performance. It combines well with other herbs and can be taken as tea or tincture or in capsules.

If you take a prescription drug that carries an aspirin warning, do not take meadowsweet, willow bark, wintergreen or other aspirin-like herbs.

MICROALGAE (Chlorella, Spirulina and Blue-green Algae)

Billions of years ago, algae covered the oceans. The first photosynthesizing organisms on our planet, they are believed to have made the earth hospitable to future life by converting carbon dioxide to oxygen, thus creating our atmosphere. Spirulina, chlorella and blue-green algae are among the world's most ubiquitous herbs and in recent years they have become among the most popular.

Not every strain of algae is edible, but the species sold as food supplements are non-toxic and rich in chlorophyll, amino acids, vitamins, minerals and protein. Proponents believe microalgae can solve the world's hunger problems, cure AIDS and cancer, treat radiation poisoning and feed astronauts in outer space in addition to more mundane tasks like lowering cholesterol, making joints more limber, detoxifying the body and increasing physical and mental energy.

Spirulina, named for its cell's spiral shape, is the only microalgae visible to the naked eye. Spirulina has become popular with vegetarians, athletes, expectant mothers, senior citizens and others who want to improve or maintain their health. First studied by scientists in the 1940s, spirulina was found to contain 65 to 70 percent protein, the eight essential amino acids, abundant vitamin B12 and other nutrients.

Chlorella, another ancient single-celled algae, derives its name from its high chlorophyll content. Chlorophyll repairs cells, increases hemoglobin in the blood and speeds cell growth. Rediscovered in the last 50 years, chlorella has its own enthusiastic supporters, who point to scientific evidence and clinical experience indicating benefits similar to those shown for spirulina.

Blue-green algae, the popular name for a strain of *Aphanizaomenon*, grows on lakes and ponds. Like spirulina and chlorella, blue-green algae contains chlorophyll, vitamins, minerals, protein, amino acids and other nutrients. Enthusiasts credit blue-green algae with curing everything from cancer to chronic fatigue syndrome, allergies, headaches, wrinkles, asthma, arthritis and AIDS—testimonials much like the exaggerated claims made for spirulina 15 years ago.

Holistic practitioners use microalgae in the treatment of arthritis, rheumatism, gout and other inflammatory diseases, constitutional weakness, anemia, memory problems, low blood sugar, poor eyesight, skin conditions, high cholesterol and blood pressure, heavy metal poisoning, allergies, ulcers and tumors. Even if the algae doesn't cure an illness, it offers important nutritional support that is easy for most people to absorb, even when digestion is impaired.

Most health practitioners recommend taking 2 to

5 grams per day for maintenance and prevention and 5 to 10 grams per day for the treatment of most conditions. For chronic arthritis, start with small doses and increase gradually. Improvement is often apparent within one to three months. Discontinue use if you experience nausea or any unpleasant side effect.

MUSTARD (*Brassica alba* or *B. nigra*)

This well-known culinary herb not only whets the appetite, it has stimulating external applications as well. Mustard poultices or plasters are a traditional treatment for chest cold congestion and muscle or bone pain. To make one, spread a paste of powdered mustard seed and water on a cloth and cover the mustard with gauze, then apply the gauze side of this mustard sandwich to the area that needs warming. Remove after a minute and check to see if the skin is reddened. If not, repeat; if so, remove the plaster and apply a thin coat of olive oil.

Few baths are as soothing to aching joints as mustard baths. See page 37 for instructions.

NETTLE (*Urtica dioica*) or STINGING NETTLE

One of the most widely used plants in herbal medicine, nettle is used to treat arthritis, eczema, anemia, gout, kidney problems, neuritis, neuralgia and respiratory conditions. Recent double-blind studies show that freeze-dried nettle effectively prevents and treats hay fever.

To brew nettle tea, pour 1 cup boiling water over 1 teaspoon dried or 1 tablespoon fresh herb. Drink 3 to 4 cups daily. The recommended tincture dosage is ½ teaspoon 3 times daily, and if you use freeze-dried nettle in capsules, take 1 capsule 3 times daily. There is no maximum dosage.

Lyme disease is a serious problem in New York State, where herbalist Pam Montgomery developed Auntie Lyme tea as an adjunct therapy in the treatment of active cases and a support remedy for those previously treated. Auntie Lyme contains nettle, red clover, comfrey, calendula, peach leaf, strawberry leaf, mint, burdock seed and milk thistle seed, a combination of blood cleansing, liver tonic and calming ingredients. Nettle tea and tincture are recommended for anyone with Lyme-induced arthritis.

In Europe, according to Rudolf Weiss, M.D., nettle tincture is applied externally to treat neuralgia, rheumatic pain, lumbago, sciatica, chronic tendinitis, sprains and similar conditions. "The effective principle in this external use is not the formic acid contained in the stinging hairs, as one would immediately assume," he wrote in *Herbal Medicine*, "but another nitrogen-free substance closely related to resinic acid, even small amounts of which will produce skin inflammation and raise weals." Nettle tincture doesn't sting the way fresh nettles do. Like other traditional European herbalists, Maria Treben recommended brushing the skin with fresh nettle (a painful experience) for relief form sciatica, lumbago, neuritis and arthritis.

OATSTRAW (*Avena sativa*)

Both oats (the familiar grain) and oatstraw (the plant's grass) are nutritive tonics for the nervous system, recommended for internal and external use in the treatment of nervous exhaustion, irritability, stress and general debility, all conditions that can accompany inflammatory disease. Though not a specific for these disorders, oats play an important supportive role. A calming tea made of equal parts oats or oatstraw, chamomile and lemon balm is both mild and effective. Oatstraw is harvested green, when the plant is young, or golden and mature. Both types are made into tinctures and sold dried for tea. Which is better? Herbalists disagree, so try both and see which you prefer. In addition to brewing oatstraw tea for drinking (1 teaspoon tea per cup of boiling water), brew an extra strong infusion (¼ to ½ cup dried tea per quart) and add it to your bath at bedtime. Oatstraw baths are delightfully aromatic and relaxing.

PRICKLY ASH BARK
(*Zanthoxylum americanum*)

The bark of the prickly ash tree stimulates circulation, though it is slower acting and more gentle than cayenne, and its tonic, antirheumatic properties make it a specific for chronic arthritis and rheumatism. It combines well with other plants and acts as a catalyst in combination with anti-inflammatory herbs. Externally, prickly ash tincture acts as a stimulating liniment for rheumatism and fibromyalgia (fibrositis).

SARSAPARILLA (*Smilax officinalis*)

Sarsaparilla, with its familiar root beer fragrance, is more than just an interesting flavor. A tonic and alternative herb, it helps tone the entire body; a diuretic, it relieves fluid retention; a stimulant, it combines well with other herbs and gently increases circulation and digestion; and an antirheumatic, it is a specific for rheumatoid arthritis and other inflammatory diseases. Brew the root as a decoction using 1 to 2 teaspoons per cup of water; drink up to 3 cups daily. The recommended tincture dosage is ½ teaspoon 3 times daily.

Sarsaparilla works well in combination with other herbs and is often featured in anti-inflammatory blends.

SKULLCAP (*Scutellaria laterifolia*)

This relaxing nervine and antispasmodic herb is considered a specific for neuralgia. In addition to relieving tension, skullcap is an effective sleep aid. It combines well with other herbs and plays an important supportive role in the treatment of arthritis, rheumatic conditions and other inflammatory illnesses.

TURMERIC (*Curcuma longa*)

Familiar as the yellow spice in curry powders, turmeric contains a powerful medicine. Its active ingredient is curcumin, which gives turmeric its intense color. Studies show that curcumin is an anti-inflammatory agent on a par with cortisone, effectively reducing the symptoms of rheumatoid arthritis. Curcumin's other actions include lowering cholesterol, preventing blood clotting, protecting the liver from toxins, improving digestion, lowering blood sugar in diabetics and fighting cancer.

Turmeric can be enjoyed in food or taken in capsules. In the treatment of Lyme disease arthritis, Michael Murray, N.D., recommends 400 mg curcurmin four times daily between meals.

WHITE WILLOW BARK (*Salix alba*)

White willow bark is considered the original, natural form of aspirin and because of its anti-inflammatory, analgesic properties, it was an ancient remedy for rheumatism, arthritis, gout, headaches and all manner of aches and pains. Willow bark contains salicin and related compounds that inhibit inflammation. Because of its similarity to aspirin, willow bark should not be taken with drugs that carry aspirin warnings, and, like aspirin, it is a short-term pain reliever, not a long-term cure for any illness.

WINTERGREEN (*Gaultheria procumbens*)

A familiar aromatic ingredient in sports rubs and liniments, wintergreen contains an essential oil that is rich in methyl salicylate, a natural aspirin, which accounts for its ability to reduce inflammation and pain. Wintergreen leaves can be heated in olive oil to create a pain-relieving lotion (see the instructions for making an oil infusion on pages 40–41) or they can be brewed as a strong tea (4 tablespoons herb per quart of boiling water) and added to bath water. Peppermint has similar antispasmodic and anti-inflammatory properties, and the essential oils of both wintergreen and peppermint are common ingredients in liniments, sports rubs and analgesic massage lotions.

YARROW (*Achillea millifolium*)

A familiar wayside plant in much of the U.S. and Europe, yarrow is also cultivated as a garden flower. For medicinal purposes, be sure to use the common weed. Bitter in taste and also useful in the treatment of indigestion, yarrow has a long history of use in North America in the treatment of painful inflammation of tissues and joints. Not everyone will respond significantly to yarrow, but for the 10 to 20 percent of arthritics who do respond to it, it will seem like a gift from heaven.

Contact dermatitis and other allergic reactions may occur in sensitive individuals. Yarrow tea has such a bitter taste that few people take it straight; it's either blended with other herbs, flavored or sweetened as a tea or put in capsules.

YUCCA (*Yucca baccata* and other species)

Native to the American Southwest, yucca has a variety of uses. Its attractive leaves and dramatic white blossoms make it a popular landscaping plant; its stems and foliage produce a coarse fiber that can be made into rope, baskets, mats, shoes, hair brushes, weather stripping and heavy brown paper; its fruit is cooked when green and eaten raw when purple; its roots can be used as a detergent for cleaning hair and washing clothes. In addition to all that, it's medicinal.

Yucca's saponin content makes it a friend to arthritics, for it reduces stress and swelling in the joints. Over 60 percent of patients tested with yucca supplements experienced diminished pain, swelling and stiffness; in addition, their blood pressure and cholesterol levels dropped, and intestinal toxicity improved as well. Yucca has no known side effects.

The standard dosage for yucca supplements is 2

tablets taken 3 times per day with meals. Results are usually apparent within three weeks, with maximum improvement after four months. Because it is so well tolerated and so effective, yucca is a popular ingredient in arthritis supplements for dogs and cats as well as people.

Bibliography

Batmanghelidj, F. *How to Deal with Back Pain and Rheumatoid Joint Pain.* Falls Church, Va.: Global Health Solutions, 1995.

——————. *Your Body's Many Cries for Water.* Falls Church, Va.: Global Health Solutions, 1995.

Burton Goldberg Group. *Alternative Medicine.* Fife, Wash: Future Medicine Publishing, 1994.

Carper, Jean. *Food—Your Medical Miracle.* New York: Harper Collins, 1993.

Douglass, William Campbell. *What They're Not Telling You About Osteoporosis.* Atlanta: Second Opinion Publishing, 1996.

Hancock, Ken. *Feverfew: Your Headache May Be Over.* New Canaan, Conn: Keats Publishing, Inc., 1986.

Hoffmann, David. *An Elder's Herbal.* Rochester, Vt.: Healing Arts Press, 1993.

Lust, John. *Drink Your Troubles Away.* New York: Benedict Lust Publications, 1981.

Moore, Michael. *Medicinal Plants of the Pacific West.* Santa Fe: Red Crane Books, 1993.

Mowrey, Daniel B. *Herbal Tonic Therapies.* New Canaan, Conn.: Keats Publishing, Inc., 1993.

Price, Weston. *Nutrition and Physical Degeneration.* La Mesa, Calif.: Price-Pottenger Nutrition Foundation, 1945.

Skousen, Max B. *Aloe Vera Handbook.* West Valley City, Ut.: Aloe Vera Research Institute, 1982.

Sobel, Dava and Arthur C. Klein. *Arthritis: What Works.* New York: St. Martin's Press, 1989.

Treben, Maria. *Health Through God's Pharmacy.* Steyr, Austria: Wilhelm Ennsthaler, 1980.

Van Fleet, James K. *A Doctor's Proven New Way to Conquer Rheumatism and Arthritis.* West Nyack, N.Y.: Parker Publishing Company, 1992.

Wade, Carlson. *Inner Cleansing: How to Free Yourself from Joint-Muscle-Artery-Circulation Sludge.* Englewood Cliffs, N.J.: Parker Publishing, 1992.

Weiss, Rudolf Fritz. *Herbal Medicine.* Beaconsfield, England: Beaconsfield Publishers, Ltd., 1988.

Appendix: Resources and Recommended Reading

Recommended Herbals

Foster, Steven, and James A. Duke. *Peterson Field Guides: Eastern/Central Medicinal Plants.* Boston: Houghton Mifflin, 1990. Superior field guide with well-documented medicinal uses.

Hoffmann, David. *The Holistic Herbal.* Dorset, England: Element Books, 1983. Popular modern reference.

Keville, Kathi. *The Illustrated Herbal Encyclopedia.* New York: Bantam Doubleday, 1992. Recommended.

Kloss, Jethro. *Back to Eden.* Loma Linda, Calif.: Back to Eden Books, 1988. Updated classic, widely used by herbalists and lay people.

Lust, John. *The Herb Book.* New York: Bantam Books, 1974. Excellent, inexpensive basic herbal.

Reader's Digest. *Magic and Medicine of Plants.* Pleasantville, N.Y.: Reader's Digest Association, 1986. Good overview, some overly cautious warnings.

Theiss, Barbara and Peter. *The Family Herbal.* Rochester, Vt.: Healing Arts Press, 1989. Introduction to European herbalism, recommended.

Tierra, Michael. *The Ways of Herbs.* New York: Pocket Books, 1983. Recommended basic herbal.

Weiss, Rodolf Fritz. *Herbal Medicine*. English transla-
tion of the sixth German edition, 1988. Imported by
Medicina Biologica, Portland, Ore. Excellent
reference.

Apitherapy (Bee Sting Therapy)
For information about apitherapy and a referral list of
apitherapists in the U.S., contact The American Apitherapy
Society at 1-800-823-3460.

Herbal Organizations
American Botanical Council, P.O. Box 201660, Austin,
Tex. 78720.
American Herb Association, P.O. Box 1673, Nevada City,
Calif. 95959.
Herb Research Foundation, 1007 Pearl Street, Suite 200,
Boulder, Colo. 80302.
International Herb Association, 1202 Allanson Road, Mun-
delein, Ill. 60060.
Northeast Herbal Association, P.O. Box 479, Milton,
N.Y. 12547.

Holistic Healthcare Organizations
Author's Note: This handbook's emphasis is herbs and
nutrition, but it's worth noting that many other approaches
to healing have helped the victims of inflammatory diseases. The following organizations offer information and
referrals.

American Academy of Environmental Medicine, P.O. Box
16106, Denver, Colo. 80216.
American Association of Naturopathic Physicians, 2366
Eastlake Avenue #322, Seattle, Wash. 98102.
American College of Advancement in Medicine, P.O. Box
3427, Laguna Hills, Calif. 92654.

American Holistic Medical Association, 4101 Lake Boone Trail #201, Raleigh, N.C. 27607.

Dried Herbs and Teas by Mail

Avena Botanicals, P.O. Box 365, West Rockport, Me. 04865.

Blessed Herbs, 109 Barre Plains Road, Oakham, Me. 01068.

Frontier Cooperative Herbs, P.O. Box 299, Norway, Ia. 52318.

Green Terrestrial, P.O. Box 41, Route 9W, Milton, N.Y. 12547.

The Herb Closet, 104 Main Street, Montpelier, Vt. 05602.

The Herbfarm, 32804 Issaquah Fall City Road, Fall City, Wash. 98024.

Island Herbs, Ryan Drum, Waldron Island, Wash. 98297.

Jean's Greens, 54 McManus Road, Rensselaerville, N.Y. 12147.

Mountain Rose Herbs, Box 2000, Redway, Calif. 95560.

Pacific Botanicals, Catalog Request, 4350 Fish Hatchery Road, Grants Pass, Ore. 97527.

Richters, Goodwood, Ontario. LOC 1AO, Canada.

Sage Mountain Herb Products, P.O. Box 420, East Barre, Vt. 05649.

Trinity Herbs, P.O. Box 199, Bodega, Calif. 94992.

Wild Weeds, P.O. Box 88, Redway, Calif. 95560.

Hypo-Allergenic Products by Mail

In addition to providing helpful products for those whose arthritis may be linked to environmental allergens, the following catalogs feature tools and equipment of interest to those who suffer from joint pain or limited mobility.

Seventh Generation, 49 Hercules Drive, Colchester, Vt. 05446-1672.

Real Goods, 555 Leslie Street, Ukiah, Calif. 95482-5507.

The Natural Choice, 1365 Rufina Circle, Santa Fe, N.M. 89750.

Self Care, 5850 Shellmound Street, Emeryville, Calif. 94608-1901.

INDEX